# *Cookbook for beginners with Diabetes*

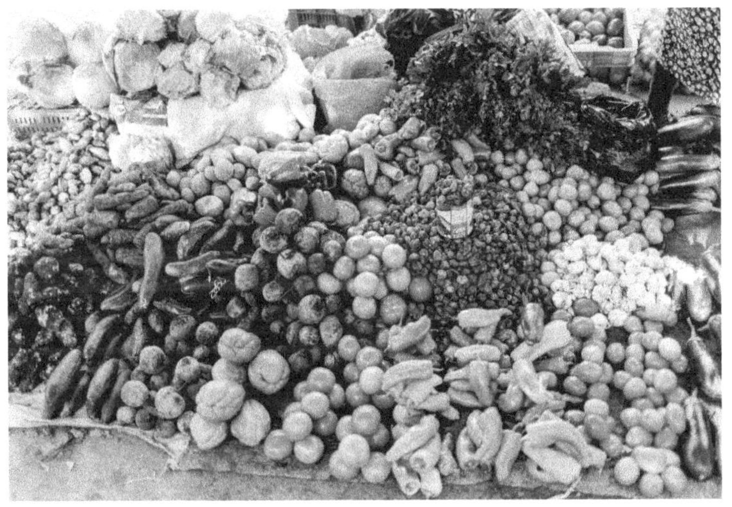

## A Comprehensive Guide for managing Diabetes through diet

### CAMILA.C.HILL

# TABLE OF CONTENT


Introduction

1. Understanding Diabetes and Nutrition

2. The Basics: Healthy Eating Habits for Managing Diabetes

3. Breakfast and Brunch Recipes

Fluffy Pancakes

Classic French Toast

Avocado Toast

Breakfast Burrito

Cheddar and Chive Scones

Huevos Rancheros

4. Snacks, Appetizers, and Beverages

5. Lunch and Dinner Recipes

Lunch Recipes:

Dinner Recipes:

6. Sweets and Desserts

7. Weekly Meal Plan Ideas

Vegetarian Meal Plan

Low Carb Meal Plan

Family-Friendly Meal Plan

Meal Prep Friendly Plan

Budget Friendly Plan

8. Tips for Meal Planning and Grocery Shopping

9. Conclusion

# Introduction

If you or someone you know is living with diabetes, then you are aware of the challenges of maintaining a healthy diet. Diabetes can be a difficult disease to manage, especially when it comes to food. However, with the right knowledge and recipes, eating healthy can be simple, delicious, and enjoyable.

The aim of this cookbook is to provide a comprehensive guide for beginners with diabetes who are looking to make positive changes to their diets. The recipes and tips in this book are designed to help you manage your blood sugar levels, eat healthily, and enjoy food at the same time.

In this cookbook, you will find easy-to-follow recipes that utilize simple ingredients and clear instructions, making them perfect for anyone who is new to cooking or looking to expand their culinary skills. The focus is on creating delicious meals that are low in carbohydrates, high in fiber, and packed with nutrients that will help you to maintain a healthy diet.

Aside from recipes, this cookbook also includes practical advice for managing your diabetes through nutrition, tips for meal planning and grocery shopping, and a glossary of terms to help you understand the basics of diabetes.

I was ecstatic when I heard that my cookbook, "Easy Cooking for Beginners with Diabetes," was finally being published. As someone who has lived with diabetes for years, I understand how challenging it can be for those who are newly diagnosed. Therefore, this cookbook is designed to make things easier for those struggling with diabetes.

When I first discovered that I have diabetes, I had no clue what to do or what to eat. It was a daunting task to figure out how to control my blood sugar levels and still enjoy tasty meals. So I started experimenting with different recipes and found ways to make healthy and delicious meals with simple ingredients. And now, those recipes have become part of the cookbook that I am sharing with others.

Each recipe in this cookbook is specially tailored to suit the requirements of diabetics. They are easy to follow and incorporate everyday ingredients that are readily available in your local supermarket. Whether you are looking for a breakfast, lunch, or dinner option, this cookbook has something for everyone.

I am determined to help people with diabetes enjoy their meals without having to worry about their blood sugar levels. I hope that this cookbook will empower those who are struggling with diabetes to take control of their health and enjoy a fulfilling life.
We hope that this cookbook inspires you to take control of your diet, enjoy healthy,

nutritious home-cooked meals, and improve your overall health and wellbeing. Let's get cooking!

# 1. Understanding Diabetes and Nutrition

Diabetes is a long-term medical condition marked by elevated glucose levels in the bloodstream. It occurs when the body cannot produce enough insulin or when the insulin produced cannot effectively move glucose from the bloodstream to cells where it can be used for energy. Nutrition plays a crucial role in managing diabetes, as what one eats can affect blood sugar levels.

**Here are some ways nutrition can help manage diabetes:**

1. Consistent Carbohydrate Intake: Carbohydrates affect blood sugar levels, and eating a consistent amount of carbohydrates at each meal and snack can help regulate blood sugar levels. This can be achieved by following a meal plan created by a registered dietitian.

2. Fiber-Rich Foods: Eating foods high in fiber, such as fruits, vegetables, whole grains, and legumes, can help to slow the absorption of glucose into the bloodstream, thereby preventing spikes in blood sugar levels.

3. Lean Protein: Eating lean protein sources such as chicken, fish, tofu, and beans can help to regulate blood sugar levels as protein is digested more slowly than carbohydrates.

4. Healthy Fats: Eating unsaturated fats, such as those found in nuts, seeds, avocados, and fatty fish, can help improve cholesterol levels and protect against heart disease, which is common in people with diabetes.

5. Limiting Added Sugars: It's important to limit added sugars, such as those found in sugary drinks, sweets, and processed foods. These can lead to spikes in blood sugar levels and increase the risk of complications associated with diabetes.

**More ways nutrition can help manage diabetes**

**1.** Glycemic Index (GI): This is a measure of how quickly different foods raise blood sugar levels. Foods with high GI (such as white bread and sugar-dense fruits) cause a larger spike in blood sugar levels compared to low GI foods (such as whole grain bread and leafy greens).

2. Balancing meals: A balanced diet that includes a mix of carbohydrates, protein, and healthy fats can help stabilize blood sugar levels throughout the day. It's best to eat small, frequent meals to prevent blood sugar spikes and to keep energy levels steady.

3. Label reading: Understanding nutrition labels is crucial for people with diabetes. Pay attention to serving sizes, total carbs, and added sugars when making food choices.

4. Sugar substitutes: Sugar substitutes like aspartame, stevia, and sucralose can be a good option for people with diabetes who want to reduce their sugar intake. However, it is important to consume them in limited

amounts and within the context of a well-rounded eating plan.

5. Alcohol: It's important to moderate alcohol consumption since it can increase blood sugar levels and interfere with medication for diabetes. It's best to stick to low-carb drinks like red wine or light beer.

6. Consultation with a registered dietician: Consulting with a registered dietician can be incredibly helpful for people with diabetes who are looking for a tailored meal plan that suits their lifestyle and health needs. Dieticians can help patients set realistic nutrition goals and make informed decisions about food choices.

In summary, a balanced diet can help manage diabetes and improve overall health. It's important to work with a registered dietitian or healthcare provider to find a meal plan that is individualized to one's needs and preferences.

# 2. The Basics: Healthy Eating Habits for Managing Diabetes

1. Eat regular meals and snacks – try to eat at roughly the same time each day and don't skip meals or snacks.

2. Choose high-fiber, low-glycemic index carbohydrates – these are digested more slowly and don't cause a rapid rise in blood sugar levels. Examples include whole grain bread, brown rice, and fruits and vegetables.

3. Limit saturated and trans fats – these can raise cholesterol levels and increase your risk of heart disease. Prefer protein sources with low fat such as fish, chicken, and legumes.

4. Reduce salt intake – try to limit your salt intake to less than 2,300 milligrams per day to help manage blood pressure.

5. Control portion sizes – use measuring cups and food scales to help you control your portion sizes.

6. Stay hydrated – drink plenty of water throughout the day to stay hydrated.

7. Limit alcohol – alcohol can cause fluctuations in blood sugar levels, so it's best to limit your intake.

By following these healthy eating habits, you can better manage your diabetes and maintain good overall health.

# 3. Breakfast and Brunch Recipes

**1. Fluffy Pancakes:** In a bowl, whisk together flour, sugar, salt, and baking powder. In another bowl, mix together milk, eggs, and melted butter.Mix the dry and wet ingredients together and stir until they are just blended.Heat a nonstick pan over medium heat and add spoonfuls of batter. Cook until bubbles form and the edges set, then flip and cook until golden brown.

**2. Classic French Toast:** Whisk together eggs, milk, vanilla extract, and cinnamon in a bowl. Dip slices of bread into the mixture and coat both sides. Melt butter in a nonstick pan over medium heat and cook the bread until golden brown on both sides. Accompany with fresh fruit and maple syrup for serving.

**3. Avocado Toast:** Toast a slice of bread and spread mashed avocado on top.Add a dash of salt, pepper, and red pepper flakes on top.Add sliced tomatoes, a poached egg, and a drizzle of balsamic glaze, if desired.

**4. Breakfast Burrito:** Scramble eggs with diced bell peppers, onions, and cooked bacon or sausage. Warm a tortilla and add the egg mixture, along with shredded cheese and hot sauce. Roll up and serve with salsa.

**5. Cheddar and Chive Scones**: In a bowl, combine flour, baking powder, sugar, salt, and baking soda. Add grated cheddar cheese and chopped chives. For the mixture to resemble coarse crumbs, incorporate cold butter by cutting it. Stir in buttermilk and knead the dough until it comes together. Pat the dough into a circle and cut into wedges, put in the oven at a temperature of 400°F and bake for 15-20 minutes until golden brown color is achieved.

**6. Huevos Rancheros:** Warm a tortilla and top with refried beans, fried eggs, salsa, avocado, and chopped cilantro. Serve with a side of rice or warm tortilla chips.

7. Banana Bread: In a bowl, whisk together flour, sugar, baking soda, salt, and cinnamon. In another bowl, mash ripe bananas and mix in

melted butter, eggs, and vanilla extract. .Mix the liquid and dry components together, and stir only until they are completely blended.Pour batter into a greased loaf pan and bake at 350°F for 50-60 minutes, or until a toothpick comes out clean.

8. Frittata: Whisk together eggs, milk, salt, and pepper. Heat a nonstick pan over medium heat and add thinly sliced potatoes, onions, and bell peppers. Cook until softened, then pour in the egg mixture and stir gently. Add grated cheese and chopped herbs, then transfer the pan to the oven and bake at 350°F for 10-12 minutes, or until set.

9. Cinnamon Rolls: In a bowl, mix together flour, sugar, salt, and yeast. In another bowl, warm milk, melted butter, and beaten eggs. Combine wet and dry ingredients and knead the dough until smooth. Let it rise for an hour, then roll it out and sprinkle it with cinnamon

and sugar. Roll up and slice into rounds. Place in the oven at a temperature of 375°F for approximately 20-25 minutes, or until they turn a golden brown color.

10. Yogurt Parfait: Layer Greek yogurt, granola, and fresh berries in a glass. Drizzle with honey or maple syrup and top with chopped nuts or coconut flakes.

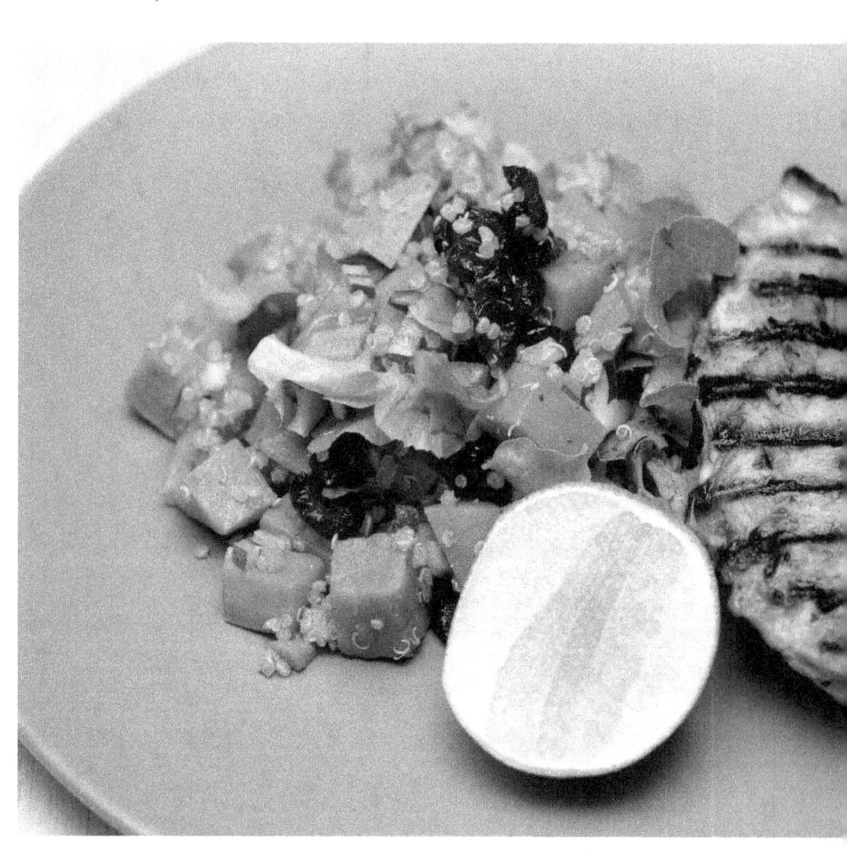

# 4. Snacks, Appetizers, and Beverages

Snacks:

1. Roasted nuts (almonds, cashews, peanuts)

2. Trail mix

3. Granola bars

4. Popcorn

5. Veggie chips

6. Cheese and crackers

7. Hummus and pita chips

8. Jerky (beef, turkey, or vegan)

9. Fruit cups or fruit leather

10. Yogurt or pudding cups

Appetizers:

1. Bruschetta

2. Caprese salad skewers (cherry tomatoes, basil, and fresh mozzarella)

3. Spinach and artichoke dip

4. Shrimp cocktail

5. Stuffed mushrooms

6. Deviled eggs

7. Cheese-stuffed jalapeño poppers

8. Chicken wings

9. BBQ meatballs

10. Flatbread pizza

Beverages:

1. Iced tea or lemonade

2. Flavored water (infused with fruit or herbs)

3. Fresh squeezed juice (orange, grapefruit, etc.)

4. Soda or sparkling water

5. Coffee or tea

6. Hot chocolate or cider

7. Smoothies or milkshakes

8. Beer or wine

9. Margaritas or Mojitos

10. Sangria.

# 5. Lunch and Dinner Recipes

## Lunch Recipes:

1. Grilled cheese and tomato soup
2. Avocado toast with egg
3. Turkey and cheese wrap
4. Chicken Caesar salad
5. Greek salad with pita
6. Tuna salad sandwich
7. Southwest salad with black beans and corn
8. Quinoa and vegetable bowl
9. Tomato and mozzarella panini
10. Egg salad sandwich.

## Dinner Recipes:

1. Chicken fajitas
2. Spaghetti and meatballs
3. Tacos with ground beef or turkey
4. Baked salmon with vegetables

5. Stir fry with chicken, beef or tofu

6. Grilled steak with roasted potatoes

7. Vegetarian chili

8. Vegetable lasagna

9. Coconut curry with shrimp or tofu

10. Grilled pork chops with rice and vegetables.

Note: Be sure to check for allergy and dietary restrictions before preparing these recipes.

# 6. Sweets and Desserts

1. Chocolate chip cookies
2. Brownies
3. Apple crisp
4. Fruit salad with whipped cream
5. Chocolate cake
6. Ice cream sundae
7. Lemon bars
8. Banana bread
9. Rice pudding
10. Cinnamon rolls.

When it comes to sweet and dessert options, it is important to consume them in moderation. Eating too much sugar can lead to negative health consequences such as weight gain, tooth decay, and an increased risk of chronic diseases such as diabetes and heart disease.

When indulging in sweet and dessert options, opt for choices that are lower in added sugars. This can include fresh or dried fruits, unsweetened yogurt, whole-grain baked goods, and desserts made with natural sweeteners like honey or maple syrup.

Additionally, it is important to listen to your body and recognize when you are satisfied. Savor each bite and don't feel the need to finish everything on your plate. By doing so, you can still enjoy sweet and dessert options while maintaining a healthy diet.
Here are some additional notes on sweet and dessert options:

1. Check the Labels – When buying sweet and dessert options, always check the labels for added sugar content. Try to choose products that are lower in added sugars or have no added sugars.

2. Portion Control – Limit your portion sizes of sweet and dessert options. It's okay to indulge in a small treat from time to time, but be sure to not overdo it.

3. Homemade is Best – Making sweet and dessert options at home allows you to control the ingredients and sugar content. You can experiment with natural sweeteners like fruit puree or stevia.

4. Be Aware of Hidden Sugars – Sugar can be hidden in many foods, including savory options like dressings and sauces. Be aware of these hidden sugars and aim to minimize your overall sugar intake.

5. Lighten Up Your Favorites – You can make healthier versions of your favorite sweet and dessert options by using alternative ingredients such as whole-grain flours, unsweetened cocoa powder, and fruits.

Remember, indulging in sweet and dessert options can be part of a healthy diet when consumed in moderation and with awareness of added sugar content.

**Note**: Be mindful of portion sizes and consider using lower sugar alternatives if needed.

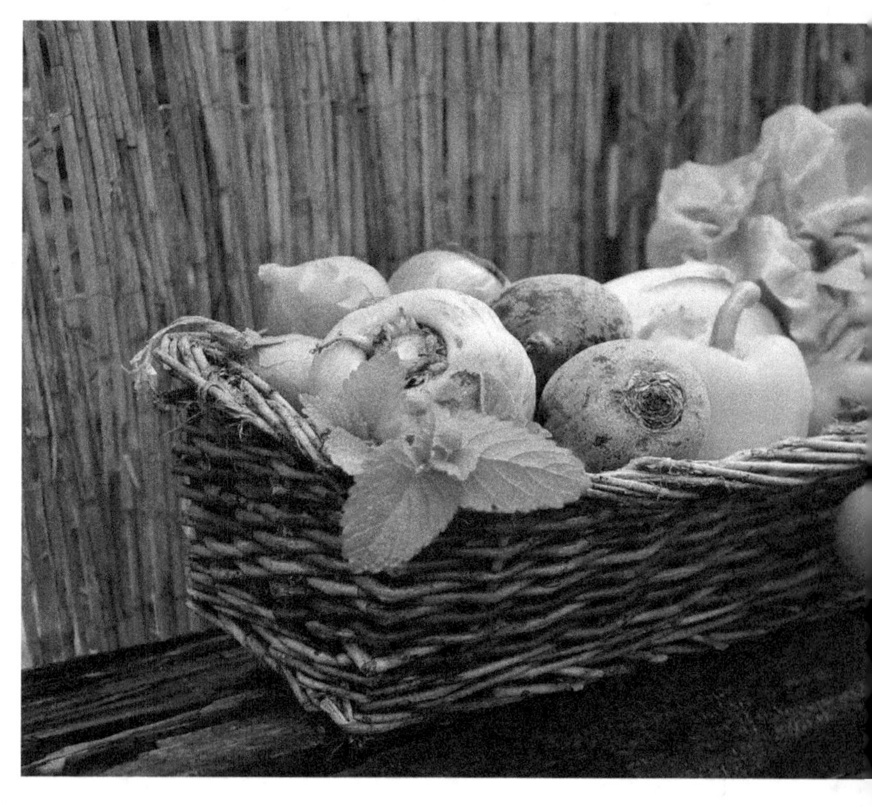

# 7. Weekly Meal Plan Ideas

Here are five different weekly meal plan ideas that could work for a variety of dietary preferences and goals:

## 1. Vegetarian Meal Plan:

- Monday: Chickpea Tikka Masala with brown rice
- Tuesday: Vegan Burrito Bowls
- Wednesday: Creamy Vegetable Pot Pie
- Thursday: Lentil Soup with Garlic Toast
- Friday: Mushroom Stroganoff with whole wheat egg noodles

## 2. Low Carb Meal Plan:

- Monday: Grilled Chicken with Roasted Brussels Sprouts
- Tuesday: Spicy Turkey Chili with zucchini noodles
- Wednesday: Baked Salmon with Roasted Asparagus

- Thursday: Grilled Steak with Mushrooms and Spinach
- Friday: Cauliflower Fried Rice with Shrimp

## 3. Family-Friendly Meal Plan:

- Monday: Chicken Alfredo with broccoli
- Tuesday: Beef Tacos with all the toppings
- Wednesday: Roasted Vegetable Lasagna
- Thursday: Sheet Pan Honey Mustard Pork Chops and veggies
- Friday: Homemade Pizza Night

## 4. Meal Prep Friendly Plan:

- Monday: Slow Cooker Chicken Fajita Bowls
- Tuesday: Broiled Salmon with Roasted Veggies
- Wednesday: Instant Pot Wild Rice Soup
- Thursday: Greek Chicken Grain Bowls
- Friday: Vegetarian Quinoa Chili

# 5. Budget Friendly Plan:

- Monday: Spaghetti and Meatballs
- Tuesday: Black Bean Tacos with Cilantro Lime Rice
- Wednesday: Three Bean Soup with Cornbread
- Thursday: Roasted Veggie and Bean Quesadillas
- Friday: Shakshuka with crusty bread

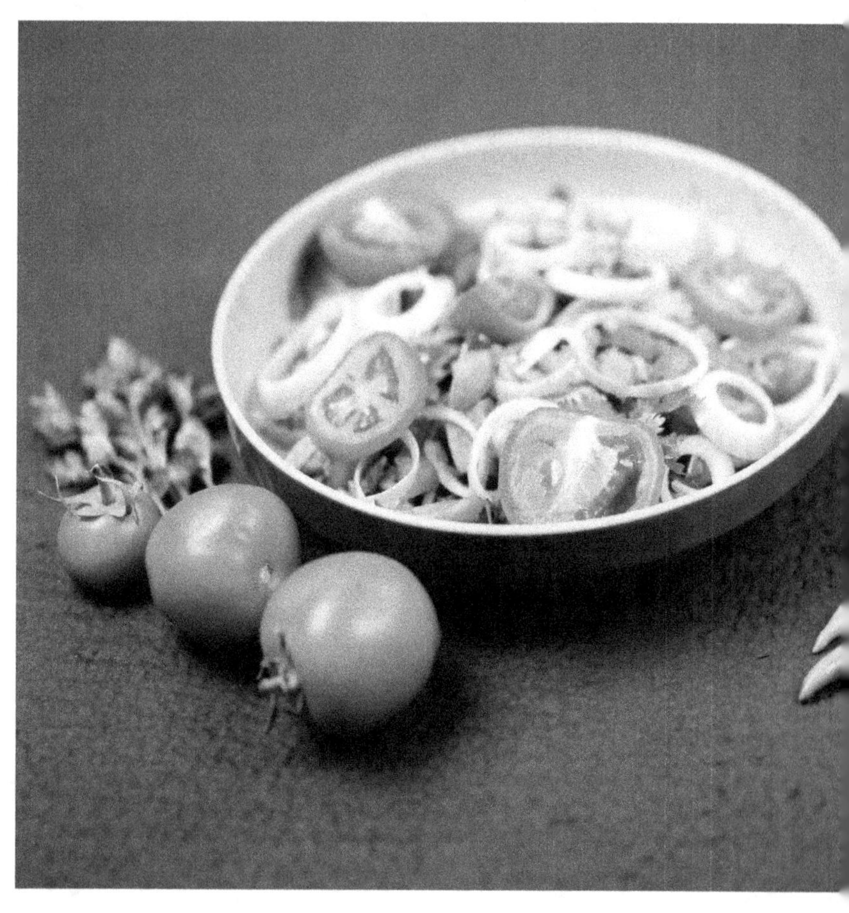

# 8. Tips for Meal Planning and Grocery Shopping

1 Start by planning your meals for the week ahead. This will give you a clear idea of what you need to buy at the grocery store

2.Create a record of all the necessary ingredients you will require. Don't forget to include spices, condiments, and other non-perishable items.

3. Check your pantry and fridge to see what items you already have on hand. Such action can assist you in preventing the acquisition of redundant items.

4. Consider buying in bulk for items that you use frequently. This can eventually lead to cost-saving.

5. As much as possible, try to adhere to whole foods.Fresh produce, lean proteins, and whole grains can help you maintain a healthy diet.

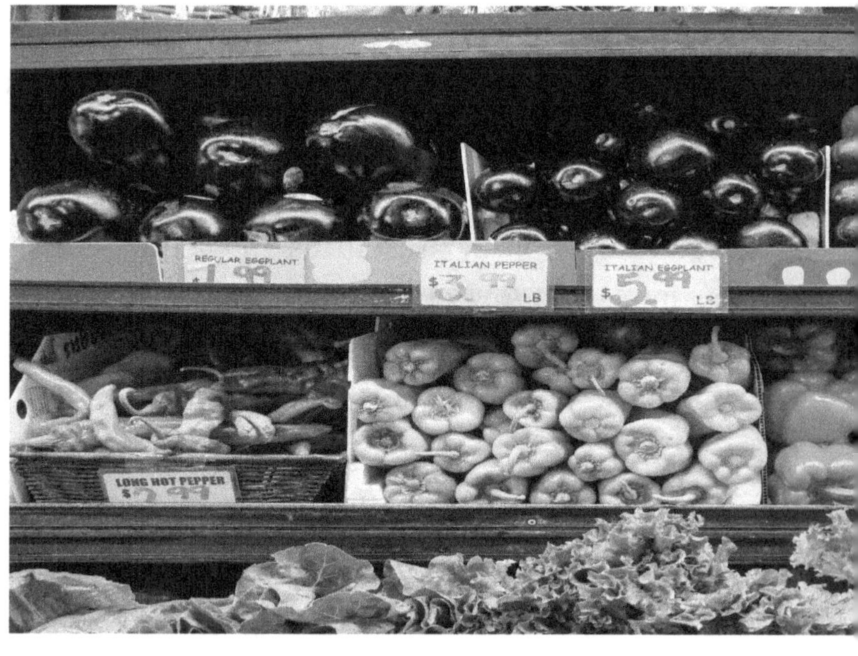
REGULAR EGGPLANT
$1.99
ITALIAN PEPPER
$3.99 LB
ITALIAN EGGPLANT
$5.99 LB
LONG HOT PEPPER
$2.99

6. Don't shop when you're hungry. This can lead to impulse buys and unhealthy choices.

7. Compare prices and look for sales. Consider using coupons or buying generic brands to save money.

8. Choose foods that can be used in multiple meals, like a whole chicken that can be used for dinner one night and the leftovers can be used in a salad or sandwich later in the week.

9. Shop the perimeter of the store as much as possible. This is where you'll find fresh produce, meats, and dairy products.

10. Don't forget to bring your reusable shopping bags and consider buying items with minimal packaging to reduce waste.

**Items that can be gotten in Grocery shopping**
1. Fruits and vegetables

2. Meat, poultry, and fish

3. Dairy products

4. Bread and baked goods

5. Pasta, rice, and grains

6. Canned and dry beans

7. Condiments and sauces

8. Snacks and treats

9. Beverages, including water, juice, and soda

10. Frozen foods

11. Breakfast items, such as cereal and oatmeal

12. Spices and herbs

13. Baking ingredients like flour, sugar, and yeast

14. Cleaning supplies

15. Personal care items like shampoo and soap

# 9. Conclusion

In conclusion, "A Cookbook for Beginners with Diabetes" is a guide for those who are new to cooking with diabetes. It is a comprehensive, practical guide meant to help people improve their health, while enjoying delicious, nutritious meals.

This cookbook provides a practical approach to cooking with diabetes. It aims to help people understand the importance of better nutrition and make healthier food choices. All the recipes are healthy, simple, and easy-to-follow. The cookbook is designed to make it easy for people living with diabetes to create healthy and tasty meals that are diabetes-friendly.

The cookbook is tailored to the specific needs of people with diabetes, helping them to maintain good blood sugar levels and manage their condition effectively. It is an essential resource that offers guidance and support to

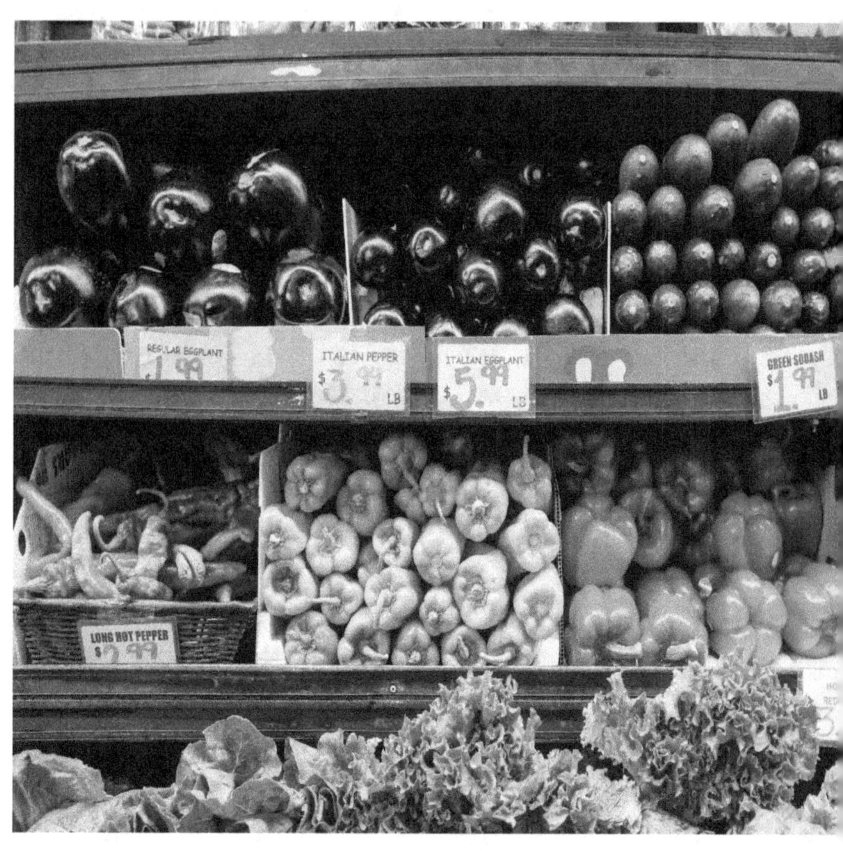

REGULAR EGGPLANT
1.99
ITALIAN PEPPER
$3.99 LB
ITALIAN EGGPLANT
$5.99 LB
GREEN SQUASH
$1.99 LB
LONG HOT PEPPER
$2.99

those who are new to cooking and managing diabetes.

Overall, "A Cookbook for Beginners with Diabetes" is a must-have for anyone who wants to start cooking healthy and delicious meals to manage their diabetes. It provides essential information on diabetes management and practical advice on healthy eating habits. It empowers people with diabetes to take control of their health, one healthy meal at a time.

## Final Thoughts

In conclusion, a cookbook for beginners with diabetes is an essential tool for maintaining a healthy diet and managing diabetes. By focusing on whole foods and balanced meals, this cookbook provides delicious and nutritious recipes that are enjoyable for everyone, not just those with diabetes. With the right knowledge and food choices, managing diabetes can be made easier and tastier than ever before.